Coconut Oil

ADISH Books

ISBN-13: 978-1494313760

ISBN-10: 1494313766

History of Coconut Oil

Coconut oil has been used in tropical regions around the world for centuries. After WWI, it was sold in Europe and the United States as coconut butter and margarine. In 1954, coconut oil began unfairly receiving negative attention during a campaign against saturated fat. The research failed to show the fact that coconut oil contains medium chain fatty acids that are extremely similar to those found in human breast milk. These fatty acids are much healthier than most saturated fats and are actually beneficial to health. In recent years, new research and thousands of personal testimonies are replacing the negative reputation once given to coconut oil. It is now commonly used both internally and externally for health and beauty.

Properties of Coconut Oil

Tropical peoples have depended on coconuts for both food and medicine for centuries. The meat, milk, oil, and juice of the nut provide rich nutrients and represent a major part of the economy and food of various cultures.

While each part of a coconut is valuable, the oil is the most remarkable food and medical ingredient. Medium chain triglycerides, also known as medium chain fatty acids, are the saturated fats that make coconut oil so unique. They are powerful antimicrobials that can prevent infections and reduce inflammation. They do not have a negative effect on cholesterol. Instead, medium chain fatty acids actually help to reduce the risk of atherosclerosis and heart disease. Coconut oil is one of the greatest sources for these rare fatty acids.

Because of the unique chemical composition of coconut oil, it is a valuable resource across the food, health and beauty industries. It can be used to treat a wound, soothe dry, irritated skin and treat acne. The oil can be ingested internally to boost the metabolism, fight infection and support weight loss efforts. These are just a few uses for coconut oil. With such a wide variety of applications, it truly is an amazing substance.

Refined vs. Unrefined Coconut Oil

Coconut oil is refined by bleaching and deodorizing. It is made from dried coconut meat called copra. During the drying process, the copra is often contaminated. It must be bleached in order to remove the contaminants. High heat then removes the oil's odor and flavor. In addition to heating and bleaching, preservatives like sodium hydroxide are often added. Sometimes, chemical solvents are utilized in order to extract the maximum amount of oil from the copra. Refined coconut oil is also often hydrogenated, adding unhealthy trans fats. Unrefined coconut oil is called "pure" or "virgin" oil. It is extracted from the fresh meat of the coconut. Two different extraction methods are often used to separate the oil from the coconut milk. Quick drying, the most common practice, hastily dries the coconut meat. The oil is then extracted using a mechanical press.In the wet milling process, the meat is pressed, resulting in coconut milk. The oil and milk are then separated by using a fermenting, boiling, centrifuge, or enzyme technique. Due to the shorter amount of time needed to obtain oil from these processes, preservatives, bleaching, and other additives are not needed. The oil remains pure with its flavor and odor intact. Many coconut oil users disagree on the best type of oil. It is generally believed that pure, virgin coconut oil is the best type since it has not been corrupted by additives, bleaching or high heat. While this is often true, if the refining process is done without the use of harmful chemicals, the difference is not as great. During the bleaching process, the polyphenols in coconut oil are damaged. They play a big part in the antioxidant effect of the oil, reducing the user's risk of atherosclerosis and cardiovascular disease. For these health benefits, unrefined oil should be used. That being said, most of the health benefits of coconut oil are in the fat. These fats remain intact throughout the refining process. For this reason, as long as it comes from a company dedicated to health and purity, refined coconut oil (as long as it is not hydrogenated) provides similar benefits to its unrefined version. Some people find the lack of odor and flavor in the refined oil preferable to the distinct, unrefined taste. Whether choosing refined or unrefined, be sure to choose a brand of oil dedicated to healthy processes and techniques.

Benefits of Coconut Oil

Coconut oil is extracted from the meat of matured coconuts. It is edible, and has a wide range of uses in the food, health, and beauty industries.

Coconut Oil for Skin

Coconut oil acts as a moisturizer, antibacterial, anti-fungal, antioxidant, and anti-microbial. Because of these properties, it's the perfect product for skin conditions of all kinds. Coconut oil contains fats that act as emollients. When used as a moisturizer, the oil quickly absorbs into the skin, providing pollutant-free, soft, healthy skin. It soothes dryness and itchiness, and can be used to treat various skin conditions like dermatitis, eczema and psoriasis. Since acne is caused by bacteria, acne vulgaris, the antibacterial properties of coconut oil make it an excellent acne-fighting solution. The oil can also eliminate acne scars by removing dead skin cells and promoting healing. However, do not leave coconut oil on the face for more than a few minutes. Doing so can clog pores and aggravate the skin further.

Coconut Oil for Hair

Coconut oil can do wonders for dry, damaged, or dandruff-ridden hair. It penetrates deep into the scalp and hair follicles to restore smooth, strong and shiny hair with body. When used as a conditioner, coconut oil prevents protein and moisture loss, protecting hair from damage. Its vitamin E and K content further promotes a healthy shine and softness. Dandruff is often caused by bacteria and infection. Therefore, the antibacterial properties of coconut oil make it an excellent tool against dandruff. It also prevents the buildup of dry skin which is another common cause of a flaky scalp. To smooth out split ends, control frizz, or give hair an added moisture boost, warm coconut oil can be applied to dry or damp hair. For dandruff control, the oil should be massaged directly into the scalp. To prevent buildup and oily hair, users may wish to wash the oil out after an hour or two.

Coconut Oil for Weight Loss

Using coconut oil to help shed pounds is not a new idea. Countless cultures, present and years long gone, in tropical regions throughout the world have used coconut oil as a main source of nutrition. Even though coconut oil has a high amount of saturated fat, those who consume it tend to live long, healthy lives. The fat in coconut oil is unlike traditional saturated fats, which helps account for the differences in the health benefits. The fats in coconuts are known as medium chain triglycerides. Your body uses these fats to produce energy. Oil can also speed your metabolism up, accelerate in burning fat and losing weight.

Instead of using butter in the morning for your toast, try spreading coconut oil on your toast. Not only does it taste amazing, but this fantastic substitution will help get your metabolism going in the morning and suppress your appetite throughout the day.

Take a tablespoon of coconut oil before heading to the gym. Since you need a good deal of energy to work out, the oil will help provide you with the boost you need, which will help you burn more calories in one setting.

After working out for the day, incorporate one to two tablespoons of coconut oil to a protein shake. Experts recommend consuming 30 grams of healthy fats after working out. Coconut oil helps to make up the healthy, fat-burning and mass-building fats.

Cook your chicken and other meat with coconut oil instead of traditional frying oils. Using this as a replacement for other saturated fats proves to be delicious and healthy. Incorporating coconut oil into your meal will help with digestion largely in part to all of the natural, healthy components within the coconut.

Take a capsule or two of the coconut oil gels with each of your meals. Try to eat five to six smaller meals per day. Countless companies offer a coconut supplement for individuals who don't want to mess with the messy oil. You will still receive all of the thermogenic, energy and fat-burning benefits with smaller amounts of the oil dispersed evenly throughout the course of the day.

Coconut Oil Benefits for Aromatherapy

Coconut oil is ideal for those who are looking for a natural perfumer while avoiding alcohol use as a carrier. Since it is the lightest of all the carrier oils, it can easily be sprayed with a pump sprayer. Thanks to its ease of use, it is also ideal for massage therapists to simply spray the lotion on to the client. Since it is has miniscule molecules, it absorbs easily into the skin and it resembles animal fat, it helps to make this an ideal oil for massages. Coconut oil leaves your skin feeling silky smooth without the oily feeling. This oil is soluble with all of the other essential oils on the market. It also works well for making soap.

It works great as a single carrier or used with other oils that are more costly for extending the shelf-life of the oil and extending the budget beyond normal reach. Since coconut oil never spoils, it has an indefinite shelf-life. Up to about 75 degrees Fahrenheit, the oil is solid. When it gets to 76 degrees Fahrenheit or above, the oil tends to turn into a liquid.

The Health Benefits of Coconut Oil

Coconut oil was long criticized as unhealthy due to its high saturated fat content. However, the oil is gaining popularity among health enthusiasts, and health professionals are beginning to think it may not be so bad after all. Once thought to cause weight gain, coconut oil is now praised as a weight loss supplement. The oil is made up of medium chain fatty acids. These fatty acids are quickly broken down by the body. Instead of being added to fat stores, they are quickly digested and used for energy.

Coconut oil further aids weight loss efforts by curbing appetite and reducing hunger. Coconut oil has also received much attention due to its ability to help those suffering from Alzheimer's and other degenerative brain diseases. Alzheimer's causes the brain to reject its main source of fuel, glucose, causing brain cells to die. Ketones, which are present in coconut oil, are easily accepted by brain cells as an alternative to glucose. Therefore, coconut oil can be used as a daily supplement to repair brain damage caused by Alzheimer's. As with all foods, coconut oil is healthy in moderation. When used as part of a balanced diet, the oil can promote a long life and healing for various diseases.

Eliminate Fatigue

Thanks to all of the saturated fats found in coconut oil, you will notice an increase in your energy levels. Countless people suffer from low energy on a regular basis, but it doesn't have to be that way for long. Coconut oil helps to cure fatigue and provide you with the energy nutrition that you need to make it through the day. Eliminate all of the mid-day fatigue by implementing coconut oil into your routine.

Anti-aging and Antioxidant Properties Abound

Thanks to the saturated fats in coconut oil of capric acid, caproic acid, caprylic acid and myristic acid, they help to counteract the effects of aging, hair whitening, sagging skin, macular degeneration and much more. The coconut oil will help leave you feeling and looking younger than ever before with all of its antioxidant properties.

Antimicrobial

All of the aforementioned acids convert themselves into monolaurin and monocaprin, which are amazing microbial and anti-fungal agents when they are acted upon by various enzymes in the body. Thanks to their derivatives, they help to protect the body, externally as well as internally, from conditions such as itches, rashes, ringworm, dermatitis, Athlete's Foot and much more. Inside and outside of your body is going to look and feel amazing thanks to the antimicrobial properties contained in coconut oil.

Candida

At one point in time or another, just about everyone has heard of Candida. Thanks to the antimicrobial properties in coconut oil, it will help to fight against this fungus and keep it from taking over your body.

Vermifuge

Tape Worms, round worms and other intestinal bugs will all be overcome through the properties in coconut oil.

Digestive Disorders

For those who are suffering with IBS, heartburn and other digestive problems, coconut oil has been found to help overcome the conditions and leave you feeling amazing. When the oil is taken on a regular basis and in the proper quantities, it will help to cure any chronic digestive problems that you have been fighting to overcome.

Cancer

Cancer is responsible for countless deaths across the country every year. Even though people are continually working to find a cure for the disease, it seems as if it is not quick enough. Thanks to all of the saturated fatty acids in coconut oil, it can help to protect your body against a number of forms of cancer. The fatty acids in coconut oil are similar to that of those in Mother's milk.

HIV

HIV has plagued the medical world for quite some time already. They have not been able to determine what needs to be done to help overcome the disease and move forward with health and healing. Recently, some rays of hope are making their way into the medical world thanks to coconut oil. Fatty acids are doing their part to help overcome the HIV virus and help restore some hope to those inflicted with the disease.

Artery Blockage

Thanks to the medium chain triglycerides found in coconut oil, it helps to lower the bad cholesterol, clear blockages and minimize the risk of heart attack. Even though there are countless comments about coconut oil and saturated fats, it works wonder for your heart.

Method for Extracting Coconut Oil

Various methods exist for extracting coconut oil. Heat, pressure and motion are some of the forces used to help separate the oil from the meat of the coconut. Depending on the method used, the oil can be extracted completely pure or it can require additional refining.

Aqueous Processing

Water is used to extract the coconut oil in this method. Separate the flesh from the coconut shell. Boil the coconut meat in water. As the meat softens and cooks, the oil escapes from the meat and is separated in the water. Coconut oil is then skimmed from the surface and gathered. Even though this method may take a bit longer, you will be able to preserve all of the oil from the coconut.

Ram Press

This press presses the oil out of the coconut with blunt force. It uses a large heavy piston with a metal tube to help filter out the oil. Once the meat is loaded into the tube, the hydraulic press helps press the meat while the oil is squeezed out of the tube and gathered together. Using this method helps to preserve the oil in its raw state, so there is no need for additional refining. This method is ideal for being able to gather the oil in its purest form, which makes it one of the main methods used.

Ghani Extraction

Ghani extraction uses a mortar system and giant pestle to help crush the meat of the coconut. Today, Ghani systems are mechanized, but the traditional presses from horses and donkeys are still used. This method helps to extract the oil in its purest form. Even though this method doesn't require as much labor, it doesn't gather as much oil as the other methods. Since this method does not provide you with as much oil as the others, it tends to be overlooked for gathering coconut oil.

Virgin Coconut Oil Extraction

Crack the coconut open and use a paring knife to get all of the coconut meat out of the shell. Grate the coconut into fine pieces; repeat until all coconut is shredded. Add ½ c. water to the coconut and squeeze handfuls of the coconut above the bowl. When squeezed, a white liquid should emerge from the coconut. You can add more water if needed. The white liquid is the coconut milk. Once you have fully squeezed the coconut and no more milk comes out of it, you can discard the coconut. Pour the liquid in a pot to cook on low. Once the liquid comes to a slow simmer, you will notice a thin layer of fat on the top of the milk. Continue boiling for another ½ hour remembering to stir occasionally. Using a ladle, skim the milk and remove the oil. Spoon the oil into a jar and seal. This method is ideal for helping to preserve all of the natural properties in the coconut.

Myths Associated with Coconut Oil

Myths about coconut oil are a disservice to humans and they are quite unfortunate. It is truly frustrating to see so many people want to destroy this amazing oil. Regardless of whether it is on purpose or by accident, speaking untruths about the oil is of no benefit to anyone. The many health blessings of this amazing oil are far too may for you to miss out on. To separate the myths from the facts, the top myths are outlined below:

Heart disease is promoted from coconut oil

Out of all the myths out there, this is the biggest one of all. Claims that coconut oil attributes to heart disease from clogging your arteries is based upon no scientific evidence. Leading detractors never ceased to spread this vicious rumor about this amazing oil until recently. Studies that made claims about coconut oil correlating to heart disease were all founded on the use of hydrogenated coconut oil. Hydrogenated oils are loaded with unhealthy trans fats, so why identify only coconut oil. Hydrogenated oils were once thought to be good for you, but the more solid the oil is, the more hydrogenated it is and the more detrimental to your health the oil is.

Animal fats and coconut oil are identical

Coconut oil and animal fats like beef tallow and lard are loaded with saturated fats. In reality, coconut oil is 92 percent saturated.

They also forgot to tell you about the molecules in coconuts being made of mainly MCFA. Vegetable oils, lard and beef fat are completely LCFA. MCFAs don't travel through your bloodstream like their LCFA counterparts. Unlike the soybean and corn oil of LCFAs, MCFA coconut oil heads right to your liver where it is changed into energy to fuel your metabolism. LCFAs and MCFAs are not like each other. Their transport, metabolism and absorption are completely different. People who consume coconut oil will lose weight, while other oils will cause you to gain weight.

Coconut oil contains a lot of cholesterol

There is absolutely no cholesterol in coconut oil. People who consume large amounts of this oil have one of the lowest cholesterol rates in the world.

The safest and best oils are polyunsaturated

In reality, nothing could be farther from the truth. Polyunsaturated oils are just the beginning of inflammatory prostaglandins, allergic leukotrienes and blood clot inducing thromboxane. When they are partly hydrogenated, they are transformed into trans fats which can be even more atherogenic. To put it simply, claiming that polyunsaturated oils are the safest and best is a complete lie. Be leery when someone tries to encourage you to ditch unsaturated fats and consume low saturated fats.

Coconut Oil Detoxification

With all of the popularity in detox and cleanses today, it can be somewhat difficult to try and find a formula that is going to help maintain vitamins in your body while still eliminating all of the toxins. Using coconut oil to detox is an exceptional choice to help cleanse your system due to its powerful and safe method loaded with healthy fatty acids. The properties help to provide you with natural energy while working to detoxify your system.

Coconut oil is loaded with fatty acids that go straight for your liver instead of heading to your body storage where all of the fat is housed. This makes it perfect for a detox cleanse because it helps to give your body the energy it needs while working to cleanse the toxins that are housed in your body tissue. Coconut oil can be found in just about any health store.

Conditions Needed for a Coconut Detoxification

Even though coconut oil has a number of different healing properties for a number of different conditions, four main reasons exist as to why people tend to use the formula. Candida tends to have a number of side effects. Since coconut oil doesn't have any carbohydrates or sugar, it helps your body to eliminate all of the toxins and qualm sugar cravings.

Fungal Infections – Jock itch and ringworm both come from disequilibrium in fungi and your body's natural bacteria. Since coconut oil is an anti-fungal, it helps to promote natural growth within your system.

Digestive – When your digestive system is not properly balanced, you may end up suffering from an upset stomach or IBS. Coconut oil can help restore your system.

Viruses – Using coconut oil will help to combat viruses thanks to the lauric acid in the oil.

How Does the Coconut Oil Detox Work?

A virgin coconut oil detox is one of the safest and most effective ways to rid the body of toxins. The oil provides natural, healthy energy during the cleansing process. To prepare for a coconut oil cleanse, it is important to begin incorporating the oil into your diet in order to let your body adjust to it.

Once you are comfortable taking 3-6 tablespoons a day, you can begin the cleanse. It is recommended that for 3-7 days you replace your regular food intake with coconut oil. Start the day with two tablespoons. Then, take up to 12 more tablespoons of oil throughout the day as desired. You may mix the oil into water, lemon juice, or plain, organic yogurt. However, it is important that you do not consume sugar during this cleanse.

The virgin coconut oil detox is great for eliminating candida, fungal infections, viruses, and digestive conditions. If you are suffering from candida, an overgrowth of yeast in the body, you may experience unpleasant side effects such as dizziness, headache, joint stiffness, and concentration problems as your body cleanses itself. This is normal and should dissipate within a few days.

Side Effects of Coconut Oil Cleansing

Some of the possible side effects experienced by those who are using coconut oil to cleanse their system for the first time are dizziness and headaches. You can help avoid this by consuming the coconut oil every day for a couple weeks before you begin the detox program. This allows your system to build the oil up and get accustomed to all of the properties it has to offer.

As with any detox, if you are taking medications or have any serious medical conditions, it is important to talk to your doctor before beginning this cleanse. In addition, if you have any serious side effects from the process, seek medical advice.

Cooking Recipes

Smoothie Recipes

If you are looking for something delectable to drink on a warm, summer day, try out some of these amazing blends to tantalize your taste buds and tickle your senses.

Banana Orange Smoothie

For those looking for a healthy treat, this smoothie blend is sure to leave you coming back for more.

Ingredients:

-1 banana

-½ c. orange juice

-3 tbsp. coconut oil

-1 tbsp. coconut cream concentrate

-3 tbsp. organic vanilla yogurt

-3 ice cubes

Procedure:

-Blend all of the ingredients together in a blender.

-To help sweeten the deal, add in five frozen strawberries to the mixture.

-You can make it thicker or thinner by changing the amount of orange juice added to the mixture.

Chocolate Coconut Smoothie

For those who love chocolate, this recipe will help deliver a tasty treat that tastes amazing and is good for you.

Ingredients:

-¾ c. raisins or dates soaked in a cup of water

-2 tbsp. organic flax seeds

-1 tbsp. shredded coconut

-1 tsp. organic cocoa powder

-1 to 2 tsp. coconut oil

-1 tsp. vanilla extract (optional)

-1 tsp. sugar

-1 chopped pear

-1 to 2 frozen bananas chopped up

-Ice cubes

Procedure:

-Soak the first three ingredients together for a minimum of 30 minutes up to a couple hours.

-Blend and begin slowly adding in the remaining ingredients. Blend the mixture thoroughly.

-Top the treat with seeds, nuts or raw cacao bins to taste.

Coconut Blueberry Smoothie

Since blueberries are loaded with antioxidants and other healthy properties, this tasty drink will help deliver a ton of nutrients all in one delicious drink.

Ingredients:

-6 oz. coconut milk

-½ c. blueberries

-½ banana

-2 tbsp. organic yogurt

-1 tbsp. coconut oil

-6 to 8 ice cubes to thicken

Procedure:

-Place everything into the blender and mix until the mixture reaches a frothy consistency.
- Pour the mixture into a glass and enjoy your tasty treat.

Coconut Pumpkin Pie Smoothie

If you are one of those who love pumpkin pie around the holidays, you can incorporate the amazing taste into a delectable treat that you can enjoy throughout the year.

Ingredients:

-¼ c. pumpkin puree

-1 banana

-½ c. coconut milk

-Dash of cinnamon

-1 tsp. honey

-1 tbsp. coconut oil

Procedure:

-Combine banana, pumpkin puree, coconut milk, honey and cinnamon in blender.

-Blend on high until the mixture is smooth and thoroughly mixed.

-While blender is in operation, pour in the coconut oil slowly.

-Pour mixture into a glass and add a sprinkle of cinnamon.

Fruity Tropical Smoothie

If you are searching for something with antioxidant, healing properties, this fruity blend will heal your body and tickle your senses. It is chocked full of different vitamins and nutrients to help provide you with a complete blend.

Ingredients:

-3 tbsp. coconut oil

-1 tbsp. coconut flour

-2 tbsp. organic honey

-1 large organic banana mashed and peeled

-1 c. unsweetened pineapple chunks

-1 c. sliced strawberries

-2 kiwis peeled and halved

-2 large mangoes cubed and peeled

-10 to 12 ice cubes for thickness

Procedure:

- In small mixing bowl, combine coconut flour, coconut oil, honey and banana.

- Mix thoroughly to ensure the oil is properly combined.

- Pour in a blender and add the remaining ingredients, except the ice cubes.

- Puree the mixture on high until blended thoroughly and continue blending for an additional minute.

- If the mix is too thick, you can add in a little water or ice and blend until the ice is crushed completely.

Raspberry and Cream Smoothie

This smoothie is creamy, filling, fruity and rich. It provides you with a natural boost of energy, which helps you get through the day and feel energized and invigorated.

Ingredients:

-¼ c. heavy cream

-¾ c. milk

-1 honey date (optional)

-½ tsp. vanilla extract

-Dash of nutmeg

-3 to 4 tbsp. rolled oats

-1 c. frozen raspberries

-1 to 2 tbsp. coconut oil

Procedure:

- Combine everything except the raspberries and coconut oil. Allow the ingredients to ask for an hour or overnight.

- Place everything into blender except the coconut oil.

- Blend until mixture is smooth while adding in the coconut oil in a steady flow.

- Pour mixture into a glass and enjoy your tasty treat.

Tropical Cocktail

Fruity, delicious, tasty and loaded with nutrients and vitamins.

Ingredients:
-1 ½ tbsp. coconut concentrate
-½ c. frozen mangoes
-1 banana ripened
-120 ml. orange juice
-1 tsp. lime juice
-3 tbsp. vanilla yogurt
-2 tbsp. coconut oil
-150 ml. water

Procedure:

- Mix the coconut cream concentrate and the water together until blended thoroughly.

- Place all of the ingredients except the oil into a blender and continue processing until it reaches a smooth consistency.

- Add in the oil and process again.

Fresh Fruity Smoothie

With all of the different fruits in this mixture, you are sure to get a load of vitamins, antioxidants and energy enriched foods.

Ingredients:

-1 c. red grapes

-2 med. peeled apples

-1 cored pear

-1 pitted peach

-1 c. strawberries

-4 oz. plain yogurt

-1 c. milk

-2 tbsp. coconut oil

-1 avocado (optional)

Procedure:

-Place everything into the blender and mix until smooth.

-If the mix is too thick, you can always add in extra milk until it reaches the desired consistency.

Muffin Recipes

First thing in the morning, you want something that is going to help awaken you and get you off to a good start. This delicious blend of ingredients found in these recipes is sure to keep you coming back for more.

Apple Coconut Bran Muffins

Moist, wholesome and delicious, these delectable muffins are great for breakfast with a glass of milk.

Ingredients:
-1 c. wheat flour
-1 c. unprocessed bran
-1 ¼ tsp. baking soda

-½ tsp. salt

-2 soy-free eggs

-6 tbsp. honey

-2 tbsp. molasses

-¾ c. milk

-¼ c. coconut oil

-1 c. grated carrots

-½ c. diced apples

-½ c. coconut flakes

-½ c. chopped walnuts (optional)

Procedure:

- Heat oven to 350 degrees.

- Stir dry ingredients together.

- In a different bowl, beat the eggs. Whisk in the honey, molasses, milk and then the oil.

- Create a well in the bowl of dry ingredients.

- Pour the liquid into your well and stir together with a whisk until they are combined.

- Add the apples, carrots, walnuts and coconut.

- Pour ingredients into muffin pan to about ¾ full.

- Bake for 20 to 25 minutes.

Banana Cacao Muffins

Potassium, protein and nutrients all around in these great-tasting muffins.

Ingredients:

Dry

-1 ¼ c. wheat flour

-7 ½ tbsp. cacao powder

-¼ c. brown sugar

-1 tsp. baking powder

-¼ tsp. sea salt

Wet I

-4 egg whites

-2 med. bananas

-½ c. plain yogurt

-1 tsp. vanilla extract

-1 tsp. stevia extract

Wet II

-60 grams chocolate chips

-3 tbsp. coconut oil

Procedure:

- Heat oven to 350.

- Whisk all of the dry ingredients together.

- In a separate bowl, whisk ingredients from Wet I together.

- In another bowl, whisk everything from Wet II until smooth.

- Pour Wet II into Wet I mix and stir until combined thoroughly.

- Pour the wet mix into the dry mix and combine everything together.

- Pour mix into muffin pan to ¾ full and bake for 35 minutes.

Banana Coconut Flour Muffins

For those who are looking for a healthy way to start their day, the potassium and antioxidants in this mixture will invigorate you and get you going.

Ingredients:

-½ tsp. baking soda

-1 tsp. baking powder

-1/8 tsp. salt

-6 eggs

-2 tbsp. melted butter

-2 tbsp. coconut oil

-¾ c. milk

-3 tbsp. honey

-1 tbsp. brown sugar

-½ tsp. vanilla extract

-2 mashed ripe bananas

Procedure:

- Heat oven to 350.

- Sift baking soda, coconut flour, salt and baking powder in a small bowl and set aside.

- In a different bowl, beat the eggs together. Add in the coconut oil, butter, milk, sugar, honey and vanilla. Whisk to combine thoroughly.

- Whisk in the coconut flour mix and the bananas until thoroughly blended. The batter should be thick.

- Divide the batter into the muffin tins and cook for 20 minutes.

Blueberry Streusel Muffins

Blueberries are loaded with antioxidants and nutrients to help cleanse your system and keep you going.

Ingredients:
-3 eggs
-2 tbsp. coconut oil
-2 tbsp. maple syrup
-2 tbsp. coconut milk
-¼ tsp. salt
-½ tsp. vanilla extract
-½ tsp. almond extract
-¼ c. coconut flour packed
-½ c. almond flour packed
-¼ tsp. baking soda

Procedure:

- Blend oil, eggs, maple syrup, coconut milk, salt and the extracts together.

- Combine the baking soda and flours to coat the fruit. Mix into the batter until you no longer have lumps.

- Pour the batter into muffin pan.

- Cook for 20 minutes at 400 degrees.

Banana Peanut Butter Power Muffin

Peanut butter has loads of protein and essential nutrients, which help to make these muffins nutritious and delicious.

Ingredients:
-2/3 c. coconut flour

-½ c. chocolate protein powder

-1 tsp. baking powder

-1 tsp. baking soda

-2 tsp. cinnamon

-1/3 c. nuts (optional)

-3 lg. bananas

-6 lg. eggs

-2 tbsp. honey (optional)

-1 tbsp. vanilla extract

-½ c. peanut butter

-1/3 c. coconut oil

Procedure:

- Preheat oven to 350.

- Mix together the dry ingredients except for the nuts.

- Blend the wet ingredients in a mixer or blender.

- Add the oil in slowly.

- Pour the wet mix into the dry mix.

- If using nuts, go ahead and fold them in.

- Allow the mix to settle for five minutes.

- Pour the mix into the muffin pan.

- Bake for 25 to 30 minutes.

Cherry Muffins

Cherries and coconut oil combine to help provide you with an abundance of energy all in one fabulous treat in the morning.

Ingredients:

-2 c. white wheat flour

-2 tsp. baking powder

-½ tsp. salt

-1 c. sour cream

-1 egg

-1 tbsp. coconut cream concentrate with water added to equal 2 to 4 tbsp.

-9 oz. jar cherry jam

Procedure:

- Preheat oven to 250 degrees.

- Grease muffin pans with coconut oil.

- Mix the dry ingredients in a large bowl.

- In a separate bowl, mix all of the wet ingredients.

- Stir your wet ingredients into your dry ingredients.

- Pour half of the batter into all of the muffin cups. Top with a tbsp. of jam. Continue filling the muffin cups with the remaining batter.

- Bake for 20 to 30 minutes.

Lunch Recipes

Depending on what your taste preferences are, you will find a number of different dishes that will help fill your stomach and tickle your taste buds all at the same time.

Coconut Chicken Salad

Protein, vitamins, minerals and antioxidants abound in this delicious dish to help fill you up at lunchtime.

Ingredients:
-1 whole chicken
-1/3 c. walnuts
-¼ c. apple chopped, but not peeled
-Dash of black pepper
-Dash of cayenne pepper
-2 pinches of celery seed
-Celery salt to season
-2 to 3 tbsp. coconut mayonnaise
-1 to 2 tbsp. mustard
-½ lg. chopped dill pickle
-¼ diced onion
-1 tbsp. dried parsley

Procedure:

- Boil the chicken in a large pot with water. Once the meat is cooked, pull the chicken out and allow it to cool. Remove the meat off the bones. Put the skin and bones back into the pot to create a chicken stock.

- Cut up the meat and use one to two cups of the meat to make a chicken salad. Save the remaining meat to form your soup.

- Mix everything together in a medium bowl. Adjust seasonings to taste.

Pumpkin Curry Soup

Help burn off fat with this tasty blend of ingredients in one scrumptious soup.

Ingredients:

-2 tbsp. coconut oil

-1 tbsp. curry powder

-1 tsp. powdered ginger

-1 tsp. cumin seeds

-½ tsp. red pepper flakes

-4 minced garlic cloves

-3 ½ c. pumpkin puree

-2 c. soup stock

-2 c. coconut milk

-Salt for seasoning

Procedure:

- Heat oil in soup pan on medium.

- Add ginger, curry, red pepper flakes and cumin.

- Stir for a few minutes until the seasonings become fragrant. Don't walk away or the mix could burn and you will have to start over.

- Add garlic and continue to stir. Avoid letting the garlic brown or its flavor will overpower the soup.

- Pour soup stock into the mixture and continue stirring. Make sure to loosen anything sticking to the pot.

- Put pumpkin puree into blender and add soup stock. Blend well

- Warm coconut milk in soup pan and add everything back in together.

Creamy Chicken Soup

Protein, herbs and spices help create this tasty treat that will help to leave you feeling fuller longer.

Ingredients:
-3 lbs. chicken cooked and shredded

-1 tbsp. coconut oil

-1 chopped onion

-4 garlic cloves

-¼ to ½ c. butter

-1/8 to ½ c. coconut flour

-2 c. chicken stock

-16 oz. stewed tomatoes

-2 chopped zucchini

-2 chopped yellow squash

-2 chopped carrots

-2 chopped celery

-14 oz. milk

-Avocado

-Cilantro

Procedure:

- Melt coconut oil and cook the onion until it softens. Add in the garlic and cook a little longer.

- Add in butter and flour slowly to help create a paste. The more of the ingredients you add, the thicker the soup is going to be.

- Whisk in the chicken stock. If the mix is too thick, add more stock.

- Add all of the vegetables and chicken to the mix. Season with salt, pepper, thyme, sage, oregano and so on.

- Allow to simmer for at least 30 minutes.

Chicken Nuggets

Enjoy consuming a meal composed of mainly protein with this fabulous dish.

Ingredients:

-2 lbs. chicken

-½ tsp. garlic powder

-½ tsp. onion powder

-1 tsp. crushed red pepper flakes

-2 tsp. chili powder

-1 tsp. salt

-Pepper

-2 eggs

-1 c. breadcrumbs

-Coconut oil

Procedure:

Mix everything together except for the coconut oil until thoroughly combined. Add additional breadcrumbs is it looks too sticky. Heat the coconut oil on medium and drop the chicken mix into the pan in the shape of nuggets. Continue cooking until the outer shell is brown on both sides.

Coconut Corn Cakes

This gentle dish will help to fill you up and provide you with a variety of different minerals, vitamins, nutrients and antioxidants.

Ingredients:
-1 c. sweet corn
¼ c. chives chopped
-2 eggs
-2 tbsp. coconut oil
-¼ c. coconut flour
-¼ c. corn masa flour
-½ tsp. salt
-¼ tsp. pepper

Procedure:

- In a food processor, whirl ¾ of the corn and the chives until they arc slightly pureed.

- Put ingredients into a different container and add the eggs and 2 tbsp. coconut oil.

- Combine thoroughly.

- Add cornmeal, salt, pepper and coconut flour.

- Continue to mix thoroughly, but not too hard.

- Heat remaining oil on medium heat.

- Place large spoons of batter into the skillet.

- Flatten them gently and continue cooking.

- Flip and repeat cooking.

Coconut Napa Cabbage Salad

Cabbage has been said to be one of the best vegetables for you for quite some time now thanks to its host of health benefits.

Ingredients:

-1 sm. head cabbage

-¼ c. coconut oil

-¾ c. almonds slivered

-½ c. sesame seeds

-1 c. shredded coconut

Dressing Ingredients:

-¼ c. coconut oil

-¼ c. coconut vinegar water

-¼ c. candied ginger chopped

-2 tbsp. whole sugar

-4 tsp. soy sauce fermented

Procedure:

- Wash the napa cabbage and chop it up.

- Melt coconut oil on medium heat.

- Add sesame seeds and almonds.

- Stir until the seeds begin to turn brown.

- Add coconut.

- Continue to stir until the coconut begins browning.

- Remove from heat and allow to cool.

- Mix dressing ingredients in a bowl.

- Toss the cabbage along with the dressing.

- Toss everything together with the cooled but mixture.

Dinner Recipes

When it comes time to enjoy dinner, you will love some of the fabulous recipes found here that incorporate coconut oil into the dish.

Apple Chicken Stir Fry

Vegetables and coconut oil help to bring this dish to life. Loaded with nutrients and vitamins, this dish is sure to help fuel your appetite for quite some time.

Ingredients:
-4 lg. chicken breasts
-2 red apples
-½ c. coconut oil
-1 tbsp. sesame oil

-¼ c. honey

-1 tbsp. shredded ginger

-2 c. mushroom slices

-Salt and pepper

-Chopped green onions

-2 to 3 c. steamed rice

Procedure:

- Cut the apples and chicken into chunks and place aside.

- Sauté the honey, oils, ginger, chicken and apples until the chicken is thoroughly cooked, which is normally eight minutes. The apples should be tender by the time this step is completed.

- Add mushrooms and season to taste.

- Sauté for an additional five minutes until mushrooms are thoroughly cooked.

- Serve the dish on a bed of rice and garnish with the green onions.

Cheesy Fried Rice

Calcium, vitamins and nutrients abound in this tasty treat. Not only is it delicious, but it has a wealth of nutritional value to help boost energy and leave you feeling fuller longer.

Ingredients:

-2 eggs

-4 tbsp. coconut oil

-2 c. cooked brown rice

-4 oz. shredded cheese

-Salt

Procedure:

- Whisk the eggs in a small bowl and set aside for later.

- Melt coconut oil over medium heat in a sauté pan.

- Once the oil is hot, add the rice and stir-fry rice.

- Move the rice to the outer edges of the pan and pour the eggs into the middle.

- Scramble the eggs until they are almost cooked and then incorporate the rice into the mix.

- Add the cheese and continue stirring until everything is melted.

- Sprinkle with a dash of salt for taste.

Coconut Chicken and Plum Sauce

Protein, antioxidants, nutrients and vitamins are plentiful in this tasty dish. It tantalizes your taste buds with the amazing flavors and juices that bring this juice together.

Ingredients:

-4 to 6 chicken thighs with the bones in them

-½ c. coconut flour

-½ tsp. salt

-2 tbsp. coconut oil

-1/3 c. water

-3 tbsp. white wine vinegar

-1 tsp. minced garlic

-¼ tsp. crushed red peppers

-6 to 8 plums halved and pitted

Procedure:

-Dredge the chicken in the coconut flour. Make sure to coat all sides evenly.

-Sprinkle with salt to taste.

-In a skillet, heat the coconut oil on medium heat.

-Once the oil is melted, add the pieces of chicken with the skin down. Cook the chicken for four to five minutes until the skin turns crispy.

-Flip chicken over to continue browning on the flip side for an additional two to three minutes.

-Stir vinegar, water, pepper and garlic. Pour mixture around the chicken.

-Place the halves of the plums around the chicken.

-Allow the mixture to cook for 10 minutes with a cover or until such time as the chicken is thoroughly cooked.

-As the mixture cooks, the sauce will thicken. For an even thicker sauce, uncover the mixture and allow it to cook for a few minutes longer until the sauce is at a desired consistency.

-Adjust the seasonings to taste.

Coconut Milk Vegetable Stew

For a hearty meal on a cool, winter day, this stew is one of the best dinners for you to try out. It offers vitamins, minerals, nutrients and more all in one hearty dish.

Ingredients:

-4 tsp. coconut oil

-1 bay leaf

-2 cardamom pods

-1 cinnamon stick

-3 green chilies

-½ c. chopped onion

-1 c. mixed veggies

-1 c. coconut milk

-1 ½ c. water

-Salt to taste

-1 tsp. lemon juice

-Coriander garnish

Procedure:

- In a pan, heat the coconut oil. Incorporate the cinnamon, bay leaf and cardamom. Fry for a couple minutes.

- Over a medium flame, add the onion and chilies. Fry everything until it turns brown.

- Add mixed veggies and cook for a couple minutes.

- Take ½ c. coconut milk and add water to dilute the milk.

- Pour the milk over veggies in the pan.

- Add salt to taste and cover pan.

- Continue cooking until the veggies are thoroughly cooked.

- Remove pan from heat.

- Add last ½ c. coconut milk and the lemon juice.

- Thoroughly mix and garnish dish with the coriander.

-      Serve   the   dish   with   rice.

Lamb Stewp

Even though many people have heard of stews and soups, stewp is a cross between the two items. Using this fabulous recipe, you can truly have it your own way. Protein, nutrients, vitamins and minerals abound in this filling and nutritious stewp.

Ingredients:
-2 to 3 tbsp. coconut oil

-1 ½ lbs. lamb stew meat

-½ lb. lamb bones

-½ lg. sliced onion

-Coconut flour for creating a stew instead of soup

-2 lg. garlic cloves sliced thin

-1 celery rib cut into smaller pieces

-2 sm. carrots cut into smaller pieces

-2 diced tomatoes

-2 diced med. red potatoes

-Black pepper for seasoning

-1 to 1 ½ tbsp. red wine vinegar

-2 bay leaves

-2 tsp. paprika

-1 ½ c. water

-2 tsp. cumin

-Coconut flour as necessary

-Salt for seasoning

Procedure:

In a large skillet, heat the coconut oil. Trim the fat from the lamb before adding it into the pot. Add the bones.

For a few minutes, brown the bone and the meat. Continue stirring to get as much of the meat cooked as possible. Add all of the remaining ingredients beyond the second teaspoons of cumin and paprika, coconut flour and salt.

Seal the pot tightly and bring the ingredients to a boil. Turn the heat down to a low temperature and let simmer. The stewp needs to slowly simmer the entire time, but do not allow the mixture to boil. After an hour, add in the cumin and paprika. Cook everything until the meat becomes tender. Make sure to stir it a few times, but prevent the mixture from boiling.

Check how thick the mixture is and add the coconut flour to help thicken the consistency of the mixture. Add water if needed. You can also add in extra veggies if you choose. Smaller portions of wine vinegar help add a subtle tartness to the dish. Add in small amounts to enhance the taste.

Desserts Recipes

After consuming a delicious meal, top the dish off with a delectable treat to help fuel your dessert craving. Depending on your individual taste preference, you will find one of these treats to provide you with a taste that you won't soon forget.

Almond Pear Tartlets

Fruits are loaded with antioxidants, vitamins and nutrients that help promote a healthy body while fueling your energy levels at the same time.

Ingredients:
-Crust

- ¾ c. almond flour
- Pinch of salt
- ½ c. pitted dates
- Filling
- 2/3 c. almond milk
- 1/3 c. pitted dates
- ½ tsp. lemon juice
- ¼ tsp. ground cinnamon
- ½ tsp. vanilla extract
- 1/8 tsp. ground ginger (optional)
- Pinch of salt
- 1 tbsp. melted coconut oil
- 2 lg. pears cored, peeled and sliced thinly

Procedure:

To make the crust, mix the dates, almond flour and salt in a food processor. Pulsate until the items are combined thoroughly. If you notice the mixture is not combining well, incorporate ½ tbsp. water and try processing again. Divide the mix into three separate tart pans. Press the mix firmly and evenly to the bottom and side of all pans. Put the crusts into the fridge while making the filling.

For the filling, combine dates, milk, vanilla, lemon juice, ginger, cinnamon and salt in blender until it becomes smooth. While the machine is running on low, add the coconut oil and blend again until it becomes smooth.

Take the pears and put them into a bowl. Add the sauce from your blender and toss the pears to coat evenly. Remove your crusts from the refrigerator and divide everything between the pans until the crust is almost overflowing. Put your tartlets back into the refrigerator and allow them to set for a couple hours.

Buttercup Bars

For those who want a tasty chocolate treat, these nutritious and delicious bars will help provide you with a yummy treat to satisfy your chocolate cravings.

Ingredients:
- ¾ c. almond butter
- 4 tbsp. coconut oil
- 4 tbsp. honey
- ½ c. cocoa powder
- Salt to season
- 2 tbsp. chocolate chips

Procedure:

Heat 2 tbsp. coconut oil and almond butter on low to medium heat. Once everything is melted, remove the mixture from the heat and incorporate 2 tbsp. honey. Stir until mixed thoroughly. Pour ingredients into a small pan. Smooth the mixture until it forms a uniform layer. Place the bars into the freezer for a minimum of 15 minutes.

Heat the remaining coconut oil on low and add cocoa powder. Take the mixture off of the heat and add in 2 tbsp. of honey. Spread the mix onto the almond mixture in the freezer. Sprinkle a dash of salt and the chocolate chips on top of the mixture. Place it back into the freezer for an additional 30 minutes.

Frozen Banana Cream Pie

Bananas are loaded with potassium and other nutrients, which help make this treat nutritious and tasty all in one jam packed pie.

Ingredients:

-12 bananas

-1 tbsp. butter

-¼ c. coconut oil

-2 tbsp. coconut flour

-1 to 2 c. graham cracker crumbs

-4 to 6 tbsp. maple syrup

-1 c. shredded coconut

-1 pt. heavy cream

-Garnish with sliced almonds

Procedure:

- Peel, slice and then freeze 10 of the bananas that have brown spots on the peeling a day before making the pie.

- Preheat the oven to 375.

Crust:

- Simmer coconut oil and butter together until melted. Allow to cool.

- Mix oil and butter mixture into the coconut flour, maple syrup and graham crackers into a consistency that allows you to press it into the bottom of your pan. Pinch the edges where needed, but make sure the mix is not overly dry or wet. Cook for eight minutes and allow to cool.

Pie:

- Place shredded coconut into saucepan on medium and stir until it is golden brown. Remove and set aside.

- Beat the cream until it forms stiff peaks. Move away for later.

- About 10 minutes before serving, slice the last two bananas and place them onto the sides and bottom of the crust.

- Using a blender, process the frozen bananas until they are soft. Spoon your mixture into the fresh bananas and fill to almost full. Scoop your whipped cream atop the surface making peaks in the cream. Sprinkle the coconut flakes on the pie and serve immediately.

Sunbutter Chocolate Bars

Thanks to the nuts in this recipe, it is loaded with protein to help provide you with energy. Enjoy this tasty treat as a compliment to any meal.

Ingredients:

-1/3 c. coconut oil

-¼ c. sunflower butter

-¼ c. carob powder

-25 drops of stevia

-¼ tsp. vanilla extract

-Sea salt

-Sunflower seeds

Procedure:

Melt the coconut oil and combine it with carob powder, sunflower butter, stevia, salt and vanilla extract. Stir ingredients until thoroughly combined. Pour everything into a mold. Sprinkle with coconut, sunflower seeds or other nuts. Freeze.

Vegan Chocolate Truffles

For those who are looking for a tasty treat without the worry of meat products, this is one of the best alternatives from which you can choose.

Ingredients:

-8 dates soaked lightly

-4 oz. cocoa butter

-2 oz. coconut oil

-½ c. brown rice syrup

-¾ c. cocoa powder

Procedure:

Depending on whether your dates are stale or not, you may need to soak them for a half hour to ensure they will blend well. Add coconut oil and cocoa butter into the food processer. Blend the ingredients until they soften and emulsify. Add sweetener and dates and continue processing until you have a paste. Incorporate the cocoa powder and blend until thoroughly mixed.

Move your mixture into the fridge for 10 minutes to allow it to stiffen. Once the mix cools, scoop the mix and roll into small balls. Roll the balls onto a plate of cocoa powder to provide a light dusting on the balls. Store at room temperature for up to two weeks.

Tropical Bananas

Bananas are loaded with potassium and other essential nutrients, which helps make this treat tasty and nutritious.

Ingredients:
-4 bananas lengthwise cut

-½ c. pineapple puree or 1/3 c. orange juice

-3 tbsp. maple syrup

-Dash of rum

-1 tbsp. coconut oil

-½ c. coconut flakes

-½ c. pecans

Procedure:
- Preheat oven to 350 degrees.

- Use coconut oil to grease an 8x8 pan.

- Place bananas into the pan. Mix the maple syrup, rum and pineapples.

- Pour mix over the bananas.

- Melt your coconut oil and mix with coconut.

- Sprinkle atop the bananas.

- Cook at 350 for about 8 to 10 minutes.

- Sprinkle pecans over the top and serve.

Skin Care Recipes Using Coconut Oil

Whipped Coconut Oil Body Butter

Coconut oil is natural, pure and relatively inexpensive. When it comes to this recipe, you only need one simple ingredient to create an amazing blend. In a few minutes, you will have enough whipped body butter for a couple months. Not only is the mix easy to make, but your skin is going to feel amazing after applying the mixture.

Ingredients:
-1 c. coconut oil
-1 tsp. Vitamin E oil (optional)

-A few drops of essential oils to help add in fragrance (optional)

Procedure:

- Mix all ingredients in a bowl.

- Mix on high for six minutes with a wire whisk until the mixture is light and airy.

- Spoon the mixture into a glass jar and seal well.

Key Lime Whipped Coconut Oil Body Butter

This whipped blend is the perfect summertime moisturizer. Beyond smelling amazing after applying the mixture, the sweet, tangy combination of lemon and lime oil helps to brighten your mood and lift your spirits. Citrus oils boast antiseptic, antibacterial, disinfectant and antiviral properties as well.

Ingredients:

-½ c. coconut oil

-1 tbsp. olive oil

-2 tbsp. aloe vera gel

-20 drops lime oil

-20 drops lemon oil

Procedure:

- Place ingredients in a mixing bowl.

- Mix on high speed for three to seven minutes with an electric mixture. Continue checking the mixture until it is light and airy.

- Spoon the mix into a glass jar and seal tightly. If your home is warm, store the mix in the refrigerator. Otherwise, room temperature is fine for storing the mix.

Homemade Hand Scrub

Your hands are a true sign of your age, so you want to keep them looking amazing. Expensive creams are loaded with chemicals and don't provide you with soft hands, but that is not the case with this scrub. Fight dry winter skin and heal cracks with this fabulous scrub.

Ingredients:

-1 tbsp. coconut oil

-2 tbsp. honey

-¼ c. sea salt

-¼ c. organic sugar

-1 tbsp. lemon juice

Procedure:

- Mix coconut oil and honey in medium bowl.

- In a separate bowl, mix salt, lemon juice and sugar until it crumbles.

- Pour salt mix over honey mix and stir until it achieves a smooth consistency.

- Store in a small bowl or glass jar.

Coconut Oil Lotion Bar

Reduce eczema, psoriasis, soften skin, relieve flaking and dryness with coconut oil. When applied to the skin, it prevents saggy skin, wrinkles and age spots.

Ingredients:

-1 part beeswax

-1 part coconut oil

-Essential Oils (optional)

Procedure:

Heat the beeswax and coconut oil in a saucepan on low heat. Breaking the beeswax into small pieces works best. Once the mixture is melted, you can add in the essential oils. Add just a few drops to the mix.

Pour the mix into muffin tins or lotion bar molds. Allow them to sit until cooled. Placing them in the fridge will help speed the cooling process.

Coconut Oil Lip Balm

Instead of having dry, parched lips, you can nourish them with this amazing coconut blend. Supple and luscious lips await you.

Ingredients:
-1 tbsp. coconut oil
-1 tbsp. beeswax
-1 tsp. olive oil or red palm oil

Procedure:

Heat beeswax, coconut oil and olive oil or red palm oil in a boiler on low. Melt the wax and oils together. Mix well and place into a storage container. Allow the mix to cool before use.

Baby's Bottom in a Jar

Make your face feel as smooth as a baby's bottom. After applying this mixture, your skin will feel soft, smooth, supple and refreshed.

Ingredients:

-1 tbsp. coconut oil

-3 tbsp. shca butter

-2 to 3 drops tea tree oil

Procedure:

- Combine all ingredients in a bowl.

- Using the back of a spoon, squish ingredients to a frosting consistency.

- Store in a glass jar at room temperature.

Non-Toxic Eye Liner

Sensitive eyes will love the coconut blend found here. It looks beautiful and accentuates your eyes giving them a glorious glow.

Ingredients:

-2 tsp. coconut oil

-4 tsp. aloe vera gel

-1 to 2 capsules activated charcoal for black or ½ tsp. cocoa powder for brown

Procedure:

- Mix ingredients together thoroughly.

- Store in airtight container.

Mascara

Many of the mascaras today have been known to cause cancer and emit toxins into the body. Thanks to the all-natural blend of ingredients found in this blend, your lashes will look luscious and your body will be safe from chemicals.

Ingredients:
-2 tsp. coconut oil
-4 tsp. aloe vera gel
-½ tsp. grated beeswax (grate the substance first and then measure)
-1 to 2 capsules activated charcoal

Procedure:

- Place aloe vera gel, coconut oil and beeswax into a saucepan and heat on low. Continue stirring until beeswax is thoroughly melted.

- Open the activated charcoal capsules and pour into mix. Stir thoroughly. Remove from heat.

- Put mix into a small plastic bag. Push it into one corner. Cut a tiny hole in the opposite corner.

- Push the mixture through the open corner and into an empty mascara tube.

Deodorant

Make your armpits happy with this fresh scent. Eliminate all of the harmful chemicals in deodorants and smell amazing in one fabulous blend.

Ingredients:
-1/3 c. coconut oil

-2 tbsp. baking soda

-1/3 c. arrow root powder

-10 to 15 drops essential oils (optional)

Procedure:

- Combine baking soda, coconut oil and arrow root into a small bowl. Cream the ingredients to a deodorant consistency.

- Add essential oils to the mix to create a number of different scents.

- Place mixture into a small container. Apply by rubbing mix to your armpits using your fingers. Allow the mixture to set for a couple minutes to avoid smearing onto clothing.

All-Day Deodorant

For those who live in humid areas, this deodorant will keep you smelling fresh throughout the day.

Ingredients:

-3 tbsp. coconut oil

-2 tbsp. beeswax

-2 tbsp. baking soda

-2 tbsp. arrow root

-1/8 tsp. tea tree oil

-1/8 tsp. lavender oil

Procedure:

- Melt coconut oil and beeswax in a pan on low heat.

- Whisk in arrow root and baking soda.

- Remove from heat and stir in oils.

- Place deodorant into container.

- Allow the mix to cool before capping it.

Hand and Body Cream

Eliminate dry, flaky skin with this nourishing cream for your hands and body. Not only does it smell wonderful, but your skin will reap the rewards in this nourishing, non-greasy formula.

Ingredients:

-¼ c. coconut oil

-1/8 c. shea butter

-1/8 c. cocoa butter

-1 tbsp. aloe vera juice

-1 tbsp. liquid oil

-5 to 10 drops of essential oils

Procedure:

- Heat coconut oil, shea butter and cocoa butter on low heat until ingredients are thoroughly melted.

- Remove from heat.

- Add liquid oil, essential oils and aloe vera juice. Stir to combine.

- Store in canning jars or other similar containers.

Tallow Bars

Sun-burned skin will love the amazing benefits in the tallow bars. It helps provide nourishment right where you need it the most.

Ingredients:

-1/3 c. coconut oil

-1/3 c. tallow

-1/3 c. beeswax

-Essential oils (optional)

Procedure:

- Melt all of the ingredients together until they are barely melted.

- Add in the essential oils and stir thoroughly.

- Pour mixture into molds.

- Allow the mix to cool and harden.

- Pop the bars out of the molds.

Sugar Body Scrub

Exfoliate your skin and lock in moisture with this amazing scrub. It helps provide your body with the nourishment it needs to prevent dry, itchy skin.

Ingredients:

- ½ c. turbinado sugar
- ¼ c. coconut oil
- ¼ c. almond oil
- 5 to 10 drops essential oils (optional)

Procedure:

- Combine oils and sugar together.

- Transfer the mix to a container that is airtight.

Body Wash

Stop drying out your skin and start nourishing it from the outside. The body wash provides you with an invigorating scent and fabulous cleansing properties in one fabulous mix. Feel fresh, hydrated and glowing in no time.

Ingredients:
-1 bar soap
-½ tbsp. glycerin
-4 c. water
-½ c. coconut oil

Procedure:
- Grate bar soap with cheese grater.

- Place grated soap into a large pot with coconut oil, water and glycerin.

- Heat on medium until soap is dissolved.

- Once the soap is dissolved, the mix will appear murky.

- Remove from heat.

- Cover mix and allow to set overnight.

- In the morning, use a mixer to mix to a smooth consistency.

- Add additional water if needed.

- Let set for another 12 hours to check consistency.

- Place the mixture in a container of choosing.

Cranberry Body Lotion

Dry skin will be a thing of the past with this fabulous smelling lotion. Moisturize, nourish and soothe your senses with this delectable blend.

Ingredients:

-1 tsp. cocoa butter

-1 tsp. coconut oil

-½ c. almond oil

-1 tsp. beeswax

-½ c. cranberry juice

-½ tsp. glycerin

-1 tsp. honey

-1 Vitamin E capsule

-5 drops orange essential oil (optional)

Procedure:

- Melt coconut oil and cocoa butter in the top pan of a double boiler.

- Blend almond oil in over low heat.

- Using an electric mixer, blend cranberry juice, honey, Vitamin E and glycerin in a separate bowl.

- Drizzle small amounts of the warm oil mix into the cranberry juice bowl and beat rigorously.

- Continue blending and drizzling until the oil is mixed with the juice.

- Stir in five drops of oil.

Harnessing the Power of Coconut Oil in Hair Care

Coconut Oil Hair Treatment

Dry hair and scalp will benefit from the conditioning properties found in this mixture. Your hair will feel smoother, softer and less frizzy. Treat your hair once per month with this mixture.

Ingredients:

-2 tbsp. coconut oil

-2 tbsp. honey

-1 large egg yolk

Procedure:

- Warm the coconut until melted if it is solid.

- Remove from heat. Whisk in honey for a minute or two to combine ingredients.

- Separate the yolk from the egg in a separate bowl.

- Whisk egg gently and slowly incorporate coconut oil and honey to the mix. Whisk thoroughly until combined.

Scalp Treatment

Scalp treatments help eliminate flakes and promote fast, healthy hair growth. It will also help to remove any buildup of shampoo and conditioner from other products.

Ingredients:

-4 tbsp. coconut oil

-2 to 4 drops tea tree oil

-3 to 4 drops rosemary oil

Procedure:

- Combine all ingredients.

- Store in an airtight container.

Coconut Honey Deep Conditioner

Leave your hair feeling nourished, soft and tangle free with this amazing blend of coconut oil and honey.

Ingredients:

-4 tbsp. coconut oil

-2 tbsp. honey

Procedure:

- Place honey and coconut oil into a small plastic bag.

- Put the bag into a hot cup of water and allow it to warm for one minute.

- Apply the mixture to your hair.

- Wrap with a towel and let sit for 20 minutes.

- Wash hair normally.

Tropical Deep Conditioner

Not only will your hair feel soft, but it will also smell amazing with this fabulous blend. Eliminate tangles, frizz and dry hair with one simple recipe.

Ingredients:

-3 tbsp. coconut oil

-2 tbsp. olive oil

-1 tsp. lemon juice

Procedure:

- Apply a warm blend of lemon juice, olive oil and coconut oil to your head.

- Steam a bath towel and apply it to your head for 15 minutes.

- Wash hair with a mango shampoo and conditioner to help create a truly tropical experience.

Final Words

I hope you must have not only enjoyed this book but also tried few recipes for your cooking, cleaning, skin and hair care. If you want to let others know about your experience, please post your valuable and constructive reviews. Your feedback matters and it really does make a difference.

I would greatly appreciate your comment because your review is going to help me improve and update my work. If you found any error or anything you suggest to change or add in this, do let me know at ypamesh@gmail.com and I promise a quick personal response.

Your review is going to make a true experience for other readers and help them make their buying decision easier. If you'd like to leave a review then all you need to do is go to review section of book and click on "Write a customer review".

Again, thank you for your time, trust and support. Also by ADISH Books are the following books –

Essential Oils Beauty Secrets: Make Beauty Products at Home for Skin Care, Hair Care, Lip Care, Nail Care and Body Massage for Glowing, Radiant Skin and Shiny Hairs

Lemon: 50 Plus Recipes for Skin Care, Hair Care, Home and Laundry Cleaning along with Lemonade, Vegan, Curd, Chicken, Cookies, Cakes and Desserts

Scrubs and Masks: 50 Simple Natural Homemade Recipes for Glowing Radiant and Younger Skin by Exfoliation, Moisturizing and Nourishing Facial Masks for All Skin Types

Juicing Magic: 50+ Recipes for Detoxification, Weight Loss, Healthy Smooth Skin, Diabetes, Gain Energy and De-Stress